MW00710658

Insider's guide
to leading your
Medical care

INSIDER'S GUIDE TO LEADING YOUR MEDICAL CARE

HOW TO ADVOCATE FOR YOUR MEDICAL NEEDS

Gina Cuyler, MD

Copyright © 2019 by Gina Cuyler, MD

Printed in the United States of America

First Printing 2019

Interior and Cover Design: Gina Cuyler, MD

Front Cover Image: © fotomek/Adobe Stock

Author Website: https://comprehensionim.com

Library of Congress Control Number: 2019910378

Print ISBN-13: 978-1-7332808-0-8

All rights reserved. No part of this book may be reproduced in any form without permission in writing from the author except in the case of brief quotations with proper and adequate citations of the source. Requests for permission to reproduce may be submitted to the author at drcuyler@comprehensionim.com.

DISCLAIMER: This book details the author's personal experiences and opinions. The author and publisher are providing this book and its contents on an "as is" basis and make no representations or warranties of any kind with respect to this book or its contents. The author and publisher disclaim all such representations and warranties, including for example warranties of merchantability and educational or medical advice for a particular purpose. In addition, the author and publisher do not represent or warrant that the information accessible via this book is accurate, complete or current. Neither the author or publisher, nor any other representatives will be liable for damages arising out of or in connection with the use of this book. This is a comprehensive limitation of liability that applies to all damages of any kind, including (without limitation) compensatory; direct, indirect or consequential damages; loss of data, income or profit; loss of or damage to property and claims of third parties. You understand that this book is not intended as a substitute for consultation with a licensed medical professional. Before you begin any change in your lifestyle in any way, you will consult a licensed professional to ensure that you are doing what's best for your situation. This book provides content related to educational, medical, and advocacy topics. As such, use of this book implies your acceptance of this disclaimer. Although the author and publisher have made every effort to ensure that the information in this book was correct at press time, the author and publisher do not assume and hereby disclaim any liability to any party for any loss, damage, or disruption caused by errors or omissions, whether such errors or omissions result from negligence, accident, or any other cause.

This book is not intended as a substitute for the medical advice of physicians. The reader should regularly consult a physician in matters relating to his/her health and particularly with respect to any symptoms that may require diagnosis or medical attention.

DEDICATION

This book is dedicated to GOD, from whom all blessings in my life have come. With GOD, I was blessed to become a physician and have the honor and privilege of helping people with one of their greatest assets---health. Thanks to my husband, my family, my colleagues, and all my friends who have provided support and prayers in my quest to help humanity.

TABLE OF CONTENTS

PREFACE

Knowledge

The heart of the prudent acquires knowledge,
And the ear of the wise seeks knowledge.
Proverbs 18:15 NKJV[1]

What you don't know can harm you

Why didn't I know? Four years of high school, four years of college, four years of medical school, over 26 years as an internal medicine physician and I didn't know. As I sat listening to the evening news, I was shocked. Twenty people were dead. Seventeen passengers, one driver and two pedestrians all killed in a stretch limousine accident. They had hired the limousine to drive them around while they celebrated one of the passenger's birthday. What I didn't know is "that stretch limousines are modified after manufacturing and are generally not subject to the same safety regulations that are imposed on protective structures for

---

[1] Scripture taken from the New King James Version. Copyright 1982 by Thomas Nelson Inc. Used by permission. All rights reserved.

passenger cars".[2] I learned that such "oversized vehicles have been involved in tragic accidents in New York before and that in 2015 a limo carrying a bridal party of eight women crashed with a pickup truck in Cutchogue, NY, killing four people".[3] I trusted that the "system" would ensure that regulations were in place to keep passengers safe. I believed that all vehicles especially ones for hire, would have safety features in place to ensure that everyone would have all the protection from injury if an accident occurred. I didn't know that some limousines were simply cut in half and stretched without adding in the safety features. In speaking with friends in the automobile industry however, I learned that this is common knowledge amongst those in the field. Those of us on the outside simply assumed how things were done. I lacked knowledge. I was wrong. Like many others who have ever ridden in a stretch limousine, my lack of knowledge could have made me vulnerable to significant harm. That same principle applies to healthcare.

As an internal medicine physician there are many things that I know about our healthcare system. I have knowledge that is common to those working inside of the healthcare industry. However, many patients would be shocked to learn that their assumptions regarding healthcare can leave them vulnerable to significant harm. Understanding of the systems we interact with are essential for us to safely reap the benefits of the interaction.

The first step to understanding is obtaining knowledge. Knowledge requires obtaining information. But information can be difficult to pull together. Medicine is complex and can be quite

[2] Mckinley, Jesse, Shane Goldmacher and Luis Ferre-Sadurni, "20 Killed in Limo Crash in New York; Deadliest U.S. Accident in 9 years." The New York Times, October 7, 2018, https://www.nytimes.com/2018/10/07/nyregion/wedding-limo-crash-schoharie-ny.html (accessed November 5, 2018)

[3] Mckinley, Jesse, Shane Goldmacher and Luis Ferre-Sadurni, "20 Killed in Limo Crash in New York; Deadliest U.S. Accident in 9 years." The New York Times, October 7, 2018, https://www.nytimes.com/2018/10/07/nyregion/wedding-limo-crash-schoharie-ny.html (accessed November 5, 2018)

confusing. That is where this book comes in. It is written to be a resource to help you understand what is going on in healthcare, what you need to be aware of, and what you can do to help ensure that you get accurate information to make your decisions. Once you understand the healthcare system and your healthcare team, you will hopefully be in a better position to direct your medical care and advocate for your healthcare needs.

INTRODUCTION

Advocating for Your Medical Needs

Self-advocacy can be defined as the action of representing oneself or one's views or interests. In other words, it means speaking up for yourself, your views and/or your interests. Whenever I talk to people about advocating for themselves, I often hear lots of reasons why they are either intimidated or do not feel it is important to do so. The reasons that are often given to me are:

1. I am not trained in healthcare

2. I am too busy with other things

3. I might offend my healthcare provider

4. I might get a reputation as a difficult patient

5. I don't feel comfortable

6. I trust my doctor or healthcare provider

7. I would not know how to advocate for myself

8. I trust my healthcare delivery system

9. I pay others to advocate for my needs

Self-advocacy can be intimidating especially when it comes to healthcare. However, it is a skill that I believe everyone can acquire. After reading this book you should be able to:

1. Understand why self-advocacy is important in healthcare

2. Understand the differences in providers of your medical care

3. Understand how to be a better advocate for yourself and your loved ones

4. Understand why you should review your health data

5. Have tips for how to obtain and review your data

6. Understand your role in your healthcare team

So, let's get started!

HOW TO USE THIS BOOK

This book is structured to help you be able to understand the process and unseen dynamics that are occurring as you seek medical care from your healthcare team. Throughout the book you will find "Pearls" and "Advocacy Tips" designed to help highlight information that should help you be better able to communicate and advocate for your needs and/or the needs of your loved ones. At the end of the book there is a section for you to make any notes about things you wish to learn more about, thoughts or questions that have come to mind, or anything else that you wish to make a note of.

Happy learning!

CHAPTER ONE

Understanding the White Coat

The People Providing Your Care

Before I teach you how to be a better medical advocate, I want to discuss who you are advocating to. It is a common misconception that everyone providing medical care and wearing a white coat has the same qualifications. This could not be farther from the truth. Let's spend some time reviewing the training and qualifications of individuals that you may seek medical care from.

Physicians

One of the people that you are likely to encounter is a physician. Physicians can be a Doctor of Medicine (MD) or a Doctor of Osteopathic Medicine (DO). They all have a bachelor's degree from a four-year college and some will also have a master's degree and/or a PhD. They have completed four years of medical school and after finishing medical school, they will go on to do an internship or residency which can range from 3-7 additional years. Some physicians may then do a specialty for which they have to do a fellowship. Fellowships can range from one to three or more years of additional training after residency. Physicians undergo rigorous testing, must meet competitive acceptance criteria and pass numerous certifications to earn their final board certification(s).

Physician testing and licensing

Before Medical School

With respect to testing, medical students must pass the MCATs (Medical College Admission Tests) though some medical schools will consider acceptance without them.

During/After Medical School

DO students take the COMLEX (Comprehensive Osteopathic Medical Licensing Exam) and MD students must take the United States Medical Licensing Exam (USMLE) Step 1, Step 2 Clinical Skills

(CS) and Step 2 Clinical Knowledge (CK), and finally Step 3 to be licensed. After completion of their residency training, they must pass the board examination in their field of training to be considered board certified. If they choose to pursue a specialty, they will then sit for another board certification in that specialty. All of this occurs through one of the twenty-four members of the American Board of Medical Specialties (ABMS) for MDs or one of the eighteen members of the American Osteopathic Association for DOs. This information is summarized in Table 1.

Physician MD/DO

- Bachelor's Degree/4 years college, some with Masters or PhDs also
- 4 years of Medical School
- Internship/Residency : 3 - 7 additional years
- Specialists do fellowships for 1-3+ years additional training after residency
- Rigorous testing/acceptance criteria with certifications to enter and progress (MCATs, COMLEX, USMLE Step 1, Step 2 CK and CS, and Step 3 licensing exams followed by board certification and recertification through one of the 24 members of the American Board of Medical Specialties (ABMS) for MDs and one of the 18 members of the American Osteopathic Association for DOs

Table 1

Nurse Practitioner

Another clinician you may see in a white coat is a nurse practitioner (NP). A nurse practitioner is someone who became a registered nurse after being a licensed practical nurse or after completing an RN (registered nurse) program. NPs have completed 4 years of college and have earned a bachelor's degree. They must have passed the NCLEX (National Council Licensure Examination) that is developed by the National Council of State Boards of Nursing (NCSBN) or similar nurse licensing exam.

Once finished with nursing school, aspiring NPs may work as a nurse for a few years to gain some nursing experience before attending NP school. Recently however, working as a nurse is no longer a mandate. Some nurse practitioner programs allow students to graduate from nursing school and enroll immediately in a nurse practitioner program. They must complete 18 to 24 months of coursework to obtain a Master of Science in Nursing and get certified by passing an examination from a Nurse Practitioner certifying board. There are five different nurse practitioner certification boards in the United States at this time, each of which awards certifications across different population foci (role specific certification).

Table 2 lists the Nurse Practitioner Certification Boards[4] and some of the areas of certification that they cover. The areas of certifications continue to grow.

---

[4] https://www.aanp.org/student-resources/np-certification (accessed Nov. 19, 2018)

There are five different nurse practitioner certification boards in the United States, each of which award certifications across different population-foci:

American Nurses Credentialing Center (ANCC)

Acute Care Nurse Practitioner Certification
Adult Nurse Practitioner Certification
Adult-Gerontology Acute Care
Adult-Gerontology Primary Care Nurse Practitioner Certification
Adult Psychiatric-Mental Health Nurse Practitioner Certification
Advanced Diabetes Management Certification
Emergency Nurse Practitioner Certification
Family Nurse Practitioner Certification
Gerontological Nurse Practitioner Certification
Pediatric Primary Care Nurse Practitioner Certification
Psychiatric-Mental Health Nurse Practitioner (Across the Lifespan) Certification
School Nurse Practitioner Certification

Pediatric Nursing Certification Board (PNCB)

Pediatric Primary Care
Pediatric Acute Care

National Certification Corporation (NCC)

Neonatal Nurse Practitioner Certification
Women's Health Care Nurse Practitioner Certification

American Academy of Nurse Practitioners Certification Program (AANPCP)

Family
Adult-Gerontology Primary Care
Emergency Nurse Practitioner Certification

American Association of Critical-Care Nurses (AACN)

Acute Care Nurse Practitioner Certification Adult-Gerontology
Acute Care Nurse Practitioner

Table 2

Table 3 summarizes the requirements for becoming a nurse practitioner.

Nurse Practitioner (NP)

- Become a registered nurse either LPN to RN or RN – 4 years of college to earn Bachelors Degree

- Pass NCLEX examination developed by the National Council of State Boards of Nursing (NCSBN) or similar nurse licensing exam

- Work as a nurse to get some nursing experience

- Complete 18-24 months coursework to obtain a Masters of Science in Nursing and get certified by passing an exam from a Nurse Practitioner Certifying Board

Table 3

Pearl: It is important to know that physicians and nurse practitioners are not certified by the same board certification exams or certifying boards. Physicians are certified by the medical board. Nurses and nurse practitioners are certified by the nursing board. Medical students and physicians undergo more extensive training and testing than nurses and nurse practitioners to obtain their certifications.

Doctor of Nursing Practice (DNP)

Something that has evolved over the years more recently is a Doctor of Nursing Practice (DNP). This title can be very confusing because when people think doctor in healthcare, they usually think of a physician. The Doctor of Nursing Practice is a terminal degree (the highest degree awarded) for those in clinical practice and in areas that support clinical practice such as administration, organizational management, leadership and policy. The DNP prepares nursing practice scholars to translate evidence into practice to improve health outcomes. [5]

To become a DNP, you must first become a nurse practitioner and then you must complete a graduate program that lasts approximately two and a half to four years, depending on whether you attend part time or full time. Programs can be on-line with a hands-on or clinical portion or they can be in person. There is no

---

[5] https://www.aacnnursing.org/DNP/Fact-Sheet (accessed November 18, 2018)

additional board certification exam required unless it is required by the area that they choose to concentrate in. What that means is that DNPs do not have to take any other board certification exam when they become a DNP. The only board certification exam that they sit for is the one they take when they get certified by one of the five certifying bodies when they originally become nurse practitioners. This was very eye opening for me, even as a physician, because I did not understand that at present, you must think of a Doctor of Nursing Practice as a Nurse Practitioner who has obtained a PhD. Table 4 summarizes the DNP training.

Doctor of Nursing Practice (DNP)

- A terminal degree for those in clinical practice and in areas that support clinical practice, such as administration, organizational management, leadership and policy. The DNP prepares nursing practice scholars to translate evidence into practice to improve healthcare outcomes.

- Become a Nurse Practitioner

- Complete graduate program lasting approx. 2.5 -4 years depending on Part time or Full time attendance

- Programs can be on-line with hands on clinical portion or in person

- No additional board certification exam required unless required by the area they choose to concentrate in.

Table 4

Pearl: DNPs do not undergo the same training and/or board certifications as MDs and DOs. After the initial certification as an NP, there is no additional board certification required for a Doctor of Nursing Practice.

Physician Assistant

A physician assistant has a high school diploma and enrolls in a 4-year college to obtain a bachelor's degree followed by a 2-year PA program or attends an accelerated Bachelor of Science/Master of Science Program. Once they complete the PA program, they go on to take the Physician Assistant National Certifying Exam (PANCE) administered by the National Commission on Certification of Physician Assistants (NCCPA). As you can see, this is also a master's level degree. Physician Assistants are trained to work with physicians. In most states, physician assistants work under the supervision of physicians. Table 5 summarizes the PA training criteria.

Physician Assistant (PA)

- **High School Diploma**

- **4 year college Bachelors Degree followed by a 2 year PA program**
  OR

- **Accelerated BS/MS PA program - 5 years**

- **take the Physician Assistant National Certifying Exam (PANCE) administered by the National Commission on Certification of Physician Assistants (NCCPA).**

Table 5

Pearl: Physician assistants like NPs and DNPs are certified by a different certifying board than physicians.

Interns and Residents

Interns and residents are physicians. They have a medical degree from an allopathic or osteopathic[6] medical school. Interns are residents in their first year of training after medical school. Residents include interns but typically, the term is used for physicians in their second year and above after graduating from medical school. This information is summarized in Table 6.

Interns and Residents

- **Have finished Medical School and are Doctors**

- **Have a Medical Degree from an allopathic (MD) or osteopathic school (DO)**

- **Interns are residents in their 1st year of training after medical school**

- **Residents include interns but typically the term is used for residents in their 2nd year and above**

Table 6

---

[6] https://www.healthline.com/health/allopathic-medicine (accessed Nov 20, 2018)

Students

Now let's talk about students. I love teaching and working with students. They are usually so enthusiastic. They are on the path to fulfilling their dreams and their goals. You may encounter medical students, PA students, and NP students when you seek medical care. It is important to remember that students are not yet licensed or certified in their field of study. They should have everything that they do reviewed by a licensed professional. I find that the students tend to have the most time to spend with you and are usually the most outwardly excited to care for you.

Some people don't like having students involved in their care but, I think it is a great benefit because they usually look at and ask questions about everything. It is always good to watch them present your case or review the history and health data that they gathered from you, with the clinician. Some important details regarding students are listed in the Table 7.

Students

- **Medical Students, PA Students, NP students are all in training**

- **Not yet licensed or certified in their field of study**

- **Should have everything they do reviewed by a licensed professional**

- **Tend to have the most time to spend with you and are excited to take care of you**

Table 7

Advocacy tip: Ask that the review the student presents to the supervising clinician be done in your presence. This is a great way to ensure that everything that you said is communicated to the clinician.

What Do the Differences in A Provider's Training and Certification Mean for You?

We just reviewed that physicians, physician assistants, nurse practitioners, doctors of nursing practice, interns, residents, and students all have different levels of training. Training provides the knowledge that clinicians use to evaluate, diagnose, and treat patients. This knowledge is evaluated during their training and through board certifications. A medical student does not have the same knowledge as a physician who has completed a residency and a fellowship.

Some general medical problems can be easily evaluated and managed by many clinicians. However, some complex medical conditions require the involvement of clinicians with more advanced training and additional certification.

EXAMPLE 1
You have been seeing your primary care clinician for a heart issue and they decide to refer you to a heart specialist for a consultation. Ideally, the next person that you see should have more training and certification than your primary care clinician in the medical specialty you are being referred to. The clinician you see should be a residency or fellowship trained physician who is board certified in

their specialty. In this case a cardiologist would be the person with the most training and expertise in that area.

Due to a physician shortage, there is a growing movement to place patients with physician assistants and NPs/DNPs for an initial consultation at a specialist visit. While PAs, NPs and DNPs are valued members of the healthcare team, all of their assessment, diagnosis, and treatment decisions will be based upon their respective training. The specialist physician is the most highly trained clinician that you can receive a medical opinion from in a specific area of medicine. It is important to note however, that specialization in one particular area does not mean expertise in all areas of medicine. It is imperative to have a clear understanding of what your clinician is qualified to give you an expert opinion on.

Advocacy Tip : If you cannot get an initial consultation with a physician, request at the visit that your case be discussed in front of you by the PA/NP/DNP and the specialist physician to ensure that all of your history is heard and processed by the physician. The specialist opinion is only as good as the data that they are given to interpret.

You cannot assume that all clinicians working in a medical department or office have equivalent training and certification to assess, diagnose and treat your medical problems. Review their qualifications.

- Where did they complete their training?
- What medical field or specialty are they trained in?
- What board certifications have they earned AND maintained?

- How long have they been in practice?

Pearl: Remember that clinicians are individuals. Each clinician must be evaluated based on their combined training and experience. Ask about what training the clinician has had AND how much experience they have in dealing with your problem or concern.

CHAPTER TWO

Electronic Medical Records (EMRs)

Tools of the Trade

Now that I have discussed who might be providing your medical care, I want to discuss one of the major tools of the medical profession, electronic medical records (EMRs). When I first started practicing medicine back in the early 1990s, we had paper charts. Paper charts were great in some regards although they did have some downsides also. The paper chart could be reviewed quickly by flipping through the pages. I could readily access anything that I needed to review. A big downside of paper charts was that if another person had the chart, I could not use it. Sometimes the chart would be missing, or another clinician's handwriting might have been illegible. EMRs helped with a lot of that.

PROS OF EMRS

Some of the pros of EMRs are:

- All documentation is legible
- Multiple members of the healthcare team can have access to the chart at the same time
- All changes in the chart are tracked with recording of every activity that occurs
- Medical care delivered can be reviewed remotely
- The chart is never missing

CONS OF EMRS

There are some problems with accessing the EMR if you do not have any electricity or all the servers are down, but that is very rare. Let us look at some of the cons of EMRs.

Displayed Medical Information Can Be Modified

Medical Information can easily be modified by any healthcare provider with authorized access to your record. Since healthcare team members are clicking and adding information during the visit and have the option to delete information, it is possible that someone could incorrectly modify the information in your chart. It may not be intentional. They may simply have misunderstood what you said, or through a slip of the hand, they clicked the yes button when they meant to click the no button, or vice versa. Most EMRs have an audit trail and with a search, a revision history of changes can be found. This takes time and typically is not easy for the clinician to access during your visit.

Example 1 - The list displaying your medical problems and your history can be changed

You may have a certain medical problem and your healthcare provider means to enter one thing but accidentally enters something else. Numerous people may be a part of your healthcare team. You may see a specialist or a clinician who is not your primary care clinician. They may enter or delete something from a shared chart that your primary care clinician had previously entered. The primary care clinician will not know that the problem they entered into the chart has been removed if they look at your chart, or the next time they see you for a visit. Problem lists are critical in helping healthcare team members know what medical issues you have and are being treated for.

~

Example 2 - Medications lists and allergies can by changed from provider to provider

When you go to see one clinician, they may enter a dose of a medication that may not be correct. I have seen medications that were previously noted on a medication list mysteriously disappear from the list with an update or an upgrade in the EMR. Sometimes the wrong form of the medication can be selected when they are adding it to the medication list. They may list that you take the medication as a liquid when you in fact take a pill. This can cause problems later when you go to have medications refilled or if there is a question about a medication.

EMRs Make Chart Review More Difficult

It is very difficult to review the entire chart because information is stored in various locations that must load on the screen. If you have ever used a computer and have tried to use multiple programs or had to work with multiple documents, sometimes there is a little lag before the documents open. With EMRs, you usually must go to different parts of the chart for different things. There may be one main screen that might give you a summary. If you want to review all the notes in the chart or documents that have been scanned into a separate part of the chart like an archive, that can take time. That loading time and that time to go from place to place within the chart, consumes visit time. Unfortunately, in many places, visit times are very constrained. The outcome is usually that people do not review as much as they should review in the record because they do not have the time to do it. Navigating the EMR slows the process down.

Reviews Can Be Misrepresented

Medical information can be reported to have been reviewed without it actually having been reviewed. There are many insurance and regulatory mandates that clinicians review certain parts of the history, medications, and allergies in order to comply with billing and coding requirements. These reviews should be performed regardless of mandates as part of an appropriate medical evaluation. What happens is that because of time constraints or trust in the accuracy of history obtained by someone else, providers may simply click the reviewed button without reviewing and verifying the accuracy of the information that is there. This can be very problematic as inaccurate information can be carried forward or perpetuated in future encounters.

Original Work Not Required

Notes can be copied, pasted or added via a template. Using computer software or copy and paste functions, clinicians can copy portions of the last note and paste it into a new note for simplicity's sake. You will have situations where people copy a physical exam or history from a prior visit and put it into the current visit's note. They may also use history obtained by someone else and put it into their note to satisfy documentation and billing requirements. They don't always verify that the information that they are copying and pasting is accurate. Errors that exist in the chart can be propagated because of these practices.

Documentation Takes More Time

EMRs take time to document visit information in. You must get to the right location, open the correct type of note, and either dictate the note, click buttons or type to enter the information. This is different from paper charts where you simply flip open the chart and write the note. The pros and cons of EMRs are summarized in Table 8.

Electronic Medical Records (EMRs)

Pros	Cons
1. All documentation is legible	1. Information can be modified by any authorized healthcare provider
2. Multiple Members of healthcare team can access the chart	2. Problem lists and history can be changed
3. All changes are tracked	3. Medication lists, allergies etc. can be changed from provider to provider
4. Allows for oversight of healthcare providers/care	4. Difficult to quickly review the entire chart due to information being stored in various locations that have to load on the screen to be viewed
5. Chart is never missing	5. Information can be reported to be "reviewed" without actually reviewing it.
	6. Notes can be copied and pasted or templated in
	7. Take time to document in

Table 8

While the list is not all inclusive, those are some of the cons that I have encountered regarding EMRs. Taking time to review these aspects of EMRs will help your understanding as we move forward. Now we can move on to factors that influence the people you advocate to.

Pearl: There are many different types of EMRs, and the information contained in one clinician's EMR should not be assumed to be shared with another clinician's EMRs.

CHAPTER THREE

Factors Influencing Your Healthcare Providers

I reviewed the people that may provide you with medical care as well as one of the tools they may use daily, EMRs. However, there are invisible forces that impact the medical care and medical decision making that goes into the care you receive. Let's look at some of these influences.

Clinician Health: Burnout vs. Moral Injury

There is great debate about what terminology should be used to describe what is happening to clinicians, especially physicians. It is a very serious issue that is often not spoken about with patients. Some use the term "burnout" while others refer to it as "moral injury".

PHYSICIAN/PROVIDER BURNOUT

Generally defined as mental, physical and emotional exhaustion due to overwork or stress.

- "Burnout" was coined in 1970 by American psychologist Herbert Freudenberger[7]
- Rates of physician and provider burnout range from 30-65% depending on the specialty of medicine that you are looking at. Emergency Medicine, Family Medicine, Internal Medicine, and Critical Care are amongst the highest.[8]
- Usually self-reported

MORAL INJURY

Recently, there has been a shift in the nomenclature by many from the term "physician burnout" which some feel is blaming the physician for not coping with untenable working conditions, to

---

[7] Informed Health Online [Internet]. Cologne, Germany: Institute for Quality and Efficiency in Health Care (IQWiG); 2006-. Depression: What is burnout? 2012 Dec 5 [Updated 2017 Jan 12]. Available from: https://www.ncbi.nlm.nih.gov/books/NBK279286/ (accessed November 15, 2018)

[8] Linzer M, Levine R, Meltzer D, Poplau S, Warde C, West CP. 10 bold steps to prevent burnout in general internal medicine. J Gen Intern Med. 2014;29:18-20. http://link.springer.com/article/10.1007/s11606-013-2597-8/fulltext.html (accessed November 28, 2018)

newer terminology like "moral injury" by offered Drs. Simon Talbot and Wendy Dean[9] which they say is what the current healthcare system is doing to physicians.

No matter what you call it, the facts are:

- One doctor commits suicide in the United States EVERY DAY
- The physician suicide rate is more than twice that of the general population (28-40/100,000 vs. 12.3/100,000)[10]
- Poisoning and hanging are the most common methods of physician suicide
- It was reported during the American Psychiatric Association's 2018 Annual Meeting that physicians have the highest suicide rate.

Growing Physician Shortage

The growing physician shortage is projected to greatly impact how patients receive medical care in the future. The current data shows:

---

[9] https://www.statnews.com/2018/07/26/physicians-not-burning-out-they-are- suffering-moral-injury/ (accessed November 19, 2018)

[10] Anderson, Pauline, "Doctors Suicide Rate Highest of Any Profession", Mental Health News, Web MD, May 8, 2018. https://www.webmd.com/mental-health/news/20180508/doctors-suicide-rate-highest-of-any-profession#1 (accessed November 21, 2018)

- Physician demand will grow faster than supply, leading to a projected total physician shortfall between 42,600 and 121,300 physicians by 2030.[11]
- Nurse Practitioners are being utilized increasingly in primary care and specialty care.
- The American Association of Medical Colleges (AAMC) anticipates an insufficient number of specialty physicians by 2025.[12]
- Less patients will have access to physicians in the future. Physician Assistants, Nurse Practitioners, and Doctors of Nursing Practice, all of whom have less years of training than physicians, will be the first point of contact for medical care.
- Mentally, physically and emotionally exhausted physicians when accessed will likely not be at their best performance level, if current trends continue.

Who Your Clinician Works For

Let's look at who your clinician works for. I bet you thought it was just you! Ideally, your clinician would just be advocating for you. In reality however, they can be regulated and/or influenced by multiple entities.

---

[11] Mann, Sarah, "Research Shows Shortage of More than 100,000 Doctors by 2030", Association of American Medical College News, March 14, 2017. https://news.aamc.org/medical-education/article/new-aamc-research-reaffirms-looming-physician-shor/ (accessed November 15, 2018)

[12] Mann, Sarah, "Research Shows Shortage of More than 100,000 Doctors by 2030", Association of American Medical College News, March 14, 2017. https://news.aamc.org/medical-education/article/new-aamc-research-reaffirms-looming-physician-shor/ (accessed November 16, 2018)

Some of these entities are:

1. Hospitals
2. Insurance Companies
3. Pharmaceutical Companies
4. Government Agencies
5. Businesses
6. Medical Groups

Employment and business arrangements can impact:

- The amount of time spent with you
- How many patients that clinician sees daily
- Who you are referred to (when a patient is referred outside of the system or network, it is often referred to as "leakage")
- What services are offered to you
- What services are discussed with you

Things to Keep in Mind

Healthcare provider influences are significant factors that you need to be mindful of. It is important that you recognize the influences at work and how they might impact your care.

Clinician Health

The provider who you are seeing could be unable to provide appropriate medical care due to mental, physical and emotional exhaustion.

Financial Obligations

Your healthcare provider could possibly be more obligated to someone other than you. Many medical students come out of medical school with a lot of debt and are under pressure to pay off that debt. A lot of clinicians have young families, are trying to buy a house, buy a car, and raise their children in addition to paying off the loans. These financial obligations may make them less inclined to speak up or lobby for changes that benefit you.

So, what does all this mean? I believe it means that you need to learn how to be your own healthcare advocate. How do you do that? Let's get started!

CHAPTER FOUR

Preparation

Self-Advocacy Action Plan

I have given you some insight into why I believe self-advocacy is necessary. Let's see what steps you can take to get started.

Before the Visit

UNDERSTAND THE FACTS

Know your own history – you should be a master of your:

- Personal history
- Family History
- Medical History
- Surgical History

- Medication History
- Allergies

BE PREPARED

Prepare for your visit. You should have an outline of the things that you want to discuss at your appointment. Write down your questions and concerns and bring them to the appointment. Take additional paper and a pen/pencil to be able to write down the answer or plan for each item on your list.

KNOW WHO YOU WILL BE SEEING

Understand who will be providing your medical care. Try to review their credentials before the appointment. Clinician credentials and training history are usually provided on the office or hospital's website. If not, you can call the clinician's office or employer directly for the information. Remember, all clinicians are not the same with respect to experience, training, and/or expertise.

At the Visit

Check for Understanding

- Verify that what you have said has been understood. I suggest patients ask their clinician to repeat what they have said back to them if necessary.

- Repeat back to the clinician what you have been told as a summary.
- Take notes outlining what the plan and the follow-up instructions are.

After the Visit

- Make sure that the visit summary agrees with your understanding of the information presented to you.
- Sign up for access to the on-line patient portal if your provider has one. Get access to your visit notes and/or get a copy of your medical record periodically.
- Review your medical record(s) and visit notes to make sure that they accurately reflect what you have said and what you understand. Get clarification where needed and have significant errors corrected if needed.

Following these steps will help you begin to improve your understanding and participation in your medical care. Once you understand, it is easier to identify knowledge gaps. You can then formulate questions and get clarification. You can also be connected to additional resources to get the information that you need. In the next chapter, we will look at the dynamics of a medical office visit.

CHAPTER FIVE

The Medical Office Visit

In the last chapter I discussed understanding as an important part of being able to self-advocate. Communication is an important part of understanding. Miscommunication can impair your ability to understand.

Miscommunication can be defined as:

Failure to make information or your ideas and feelings clear to somebody
or
Failure to understand what somebody says to you.

When I talk about miscommunication, I always like to reference the telephone game. When I was a child, we would play a game called the telephone game. You would have one person at the beginning of a line of numerous people and you would tell the first person a story. That person would turn and tell the story that they heard to the next person in the line. The interesting thing about the game is that by the time the story got to the last person, it often did not resemble in any form the original story that had been told. Much like the communication breakdown that can happen during the game, the same thing can occur during a healthcare visit. This is why I always like to illustrate the process of the healthcare visit, that is, the process of moving through the healthcare system, as a type of telephone game which I call the "Visit Telephone Game". This does not mean that healthcare is a game. However, it has the same pitfalls in communication that the telephone game has.

The Big Picture – The Visit Overview

Let's look at the steps in the healthcare visit and what issues can arise at each step. It is important that it is understood that any miscommunication at any point in the cycle may not be noted until a future visit, a hospitalization, a chart review, or until an unwanted outcome such as death occurs. In the next few chapters, we will review each step shown in Table 9 in detail.

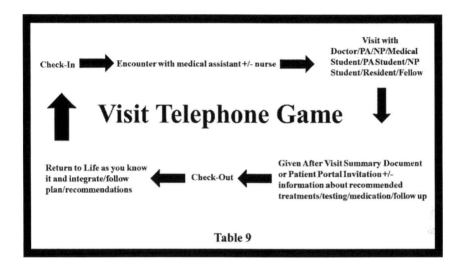

Pearl: Miscommunication or documentation errors can occur at any point in the encounter. Both can impact your medical evaluation, diagnosis, and treatment.

CHAPTER SIX

The Check-In

It is important to understand the purpose of each step of the visit so you can be prepared with the appropriate information. This understanding will also make it easier for you to identify any points in the visit where potential errors or miscommunication may occur. Let's start in Table 10 with errors that can occur when you are checking in for a visit.

Communication Errors:

Check-In ➡
- **Who you are seeing**
- **Insurance Information**
- **Reason for the visit**
- **Type of visit you are there for**

Table 10

The Purpose of Check-In

- Announce your arrival and initiate the office visit process
- Verify your insurance
- Collect signatures on regulatory and billing paperwork
- Collect your demographic information

Let's look at some of the communication errors that may occur during the check in process.

Scheduling Errors

Discrepancies in which clinician you are seeing can occur. A patient may arrive thinking their appointment is with one clinician only to be notified upon arrival that it is with a different clinician.

Example: You believe that you are going to see your primary care physician, but you are instead seeing a Nurse Practitioner or a Physician Assistant. You may also be seeing a medical student or a resident. Who you are seeing can be very confusing and at times frustrating.

Advocacy Tip: You have a right to choose who you have an appointment with. Respectfully and calmly let your preference be known to the staff. Ask to speak to the office manager or administrator if needed to discuss your options. If there has been a change in clinicians, make sure that you understand the qualifications of the clinician you will be seeing. If you have an urgent problem or become acutely ill, the best course of action is not to delay medical care. You can request involvement of a clinician with greater expertise if needed, after the initial evaluation by the first clinician you are evaluated by.

Questions you can ask:

- *Will the clinician you see be discussing your case with your physician or primary care clinician at the time of your visit?*

- *If the person evaluating you is not a physician, will your care have input from   a physician at any point during the visit?*

Insurance

Errors may occur regarding what kind of insurance you have or your insurance information. Communication errors can happen if you for example are coming in to be seen for a Worker's Compensation visit. Some practices do not accept Worker's Compensation insurance, but you may have been scheduled despite that fact and are made aware of that fact only after you have arrived. You check-in thinking you were going to have a problem addressed but are told that they will not treat you for that problem because of your insurance. This can be a very difficult situation to be in.

Advocacy Tips:

- *If you have an acute work-related problem (injury etc.), ask if they can facilitate an appointment for you with a clinician that does accept Worker's Compensation insurance.*

- *If you were to be seen for a non-work-related issue and they do not accept your insurance, find out if you can pay for the visit and be reimbursed by your insurance.*

- *Stay calm, speak softly and request assistance from the staff, the office manager, and/or your physician if needed.*

- *Call your insurance company and get help from the customer service representative with the issue.*

- *Contact human resources at your job to see if they have any resources for you.*

- *Do not let frustration prevent you from getting the medical care that you need.*

Reason for The Visit

Sometimes patients are too embarrassed to say what they are really scheduling a visit for on the phone or they do not want to take the time to tell the person scheduling the appointment all the things that they want to have addressed. As a result, they may just pick one thing to disclose or make a less embarrassing reason up. The issue is that they are not scheduled for an appropriate length of visit and that can cause problems during the visit because certain concerns require more time be allotted.

Advocacy tips:

- *Convey a brief summary of the concerns that you want discussed (headache, ankle pain, diabetes, etc.) with the person scheduling the appointment so that an adequate amount of time may be scheduled for your appointment*

- *Try to find out how long the office visit is scheduled for. If it takes you fifteen minutes just to tell your history, it will be challenging to have all of your problems assessed, diagnosed, and treated in ten minutes*

- *If the duration of the appointment seems inadequate, ask if a longer visit is possible*

Type of Visit

Issues may also occur regarding the type of visit that you are there for. Sometimes you think that you are coming in for a physical. You have saved up all your problems for your next appointment with your doctor. You have told yourself that you are going to have all your issues addressed at the physical and since it is a physical, you may not have a co-pay. You believe that you will be good as gold and right as rain when your visit is done. However, there is a miscommunication and it turns out that you are scheduled for an office visit. An office visit is not enough time for you to have all those issues addressed. Also, it can have financial consequences. Sometimes you pay a copay with an office visit but not with physicals. Sometimes, you may have to pay for the entire cost of the visit. There can be a difference in the price of an office visit and a physical. These communication failures can lead to a lot of confusion and can have financial implications. Just as important as "Reason for Visit", make sure that you understand if you are being seen for a physical, follow up visit, or sick visit (also known as acute visit). Sick visits are usually for an evaluation of one illness/problem.

Advocacy Tip: Clarify what type of appointment you are being scheduled for with the person scheduling the appointment to avoid any confusion later.

CHAPTER SEVEN

Getting Started with the Medical Assistant or Nurse

Now let's move through the encounter with the medical assistant or nurse (Table 11).

Encounter with medical assistant and/or nurse	➡	Communication Errors: • **Medications and dosages** • **Allergies** • **Medical History** • **Habits-smoking, alcohol, drugs** • **Reason for the visit**
Table 11		

After you check in, you usually sit in the waiting room until someone comes to get you. That person is usually a medical assistant or a nurse.

A common scenario is as follows. You exchange pleasantries and they take you back and start to measure your height and weight. This is followed by your vital signs (blood pressure, pulse etc.) in the exam room after additional pleasantries are exchanged. Now that you are in the room, here is where a large potential for communication errors exists.

The Conversation

Most people do not realize how important the conversation with the medical assistant or the nurse is. Usually they will sit down and chat with you while they are entering information into the computer. Now you might see them as a middle person. You might not recognize the importance they play in the care that you are going to receive that day. They will ask you if you have had any changes in your medications since the last visit and will update your information. You may say, "Yes, I started taking medication x, y, or z", and they will enter that into the computer. They may enter it however, incorrectly. They may enter it with the wrong dosage, they may enter the wrong route, or they may not have even chosen the right drug. But they entered it.

Advocacy Tip: Do not minimize the value of any conversation you have with anyone involved in your medical care. All communication has the potential to impact your care for better or for worse.

Allergies

There may be errors regarding your allergies. You may forget to mention new allergies, or they pick a wrong allergy because they could not find the exact allergy that you mentioned from a drop-down list.

Advocacy Tip: Keep a list of all your food, environmental and medication allergies. Bring a copy of the list to your appointment with you.

History

There may be errors regarding your medical history. You may mention that you were diagnosed with a certain problem and they may add that incorrectly to the problem list. Another issue is they may click the wrong button when trying to document your medical problems and click a yes or no button incorrectly for a problem.

Advocacy Tip: Keep an updated list of your history and your medical problems.

Habits

I also have seen errors when it comes to habits. Smoking, alcohol, and drug usage are all considered habits. People may accidentally put that you were a smoker when you were not, or you drank or had a substance abuse history when you did not. All of this can be done with the click of a button. It could be a result of miscommunication or misunderstanding; however, these are significant errors. In many cases, people do not realize that the wrong box has been clicked. It is not realized until they are applying for life insurance, disability insurance, or health insurance, and this information shows up at the requesting agency.

Advocacy Tip: Make a habit of verifying that your habits are noted correctly in your records.

The Chief Complaint

The chief complaint is the primary reason you are being seen. It may be the sole reason or one of several reasons for your visit. You may have lots of things that you want to discuss at the visit. However, some of those things may be personal or sensitive and you don't feel like spending time explaining all the details. Instead, you might say "I am here today for toe pain". So, the medical assistant or nurse writes down toe pain as the reason for the visit or chief complaint. They then wish you well and they leave the room. However, every part of their conversation and documentation sets the stage for the visit with the clinician.

Advocacy Tips:

- *Do not minimize the importance of the role of the medical assistant or nurse. They are gathering and updating information that the clinician will use to assess, diagnose and treat you.*

- *Be concise but clear in your conversation.*

- *Be polite and answer all questions but do not take a lot of time with non-medical chatter. Too much time spent in this portion of the visit can decrease the time you have with the clinician.*

CHAPTER EIGHT

Visit with Doctor/PA/NP/Student

The Moment You Have Waited For

Communication Errors:

Visit with Doctor/PA/NP/Medical Student/Resident/Fellow

- Medications
- History (Past Medical, Family, Present illness, Social, etc.)
- Allergies
- Reason for visit
- Diagnosis
- Treatment
- Qualifications of provider
- Plan
- Follow up
- Unaddressed Issues/Symptoms

Table 12

Now, the next person that comes through the door is going to be either a physician, physician assistant, nurse practitioner, medical student, resident or fellow. In many cases if time has allowed, they will review your chart notes before they enter the room. In reviewing the chart, they are going to be looking at what the medical assistant or nurse has just entered. The medical assistant or nurse is going to enter the reason for visit, and the clinician is going to see that reason for visit. In the clinician's mind, they are going to start allotting their time to address your concerns.

In the last chapter we used toe pain as the reason for visit. Let's look at how that would look in this scenario. After reviewing the chart, the clinician might allot most of their time for a simple reason for visit of your "pain in the toe". They may walk into the room, exchange pleasantries, sit down, and say something like, "So I hear you are having pain in your toe." You may then respond "Oh, yes. I am having pain in the toe". They will proceed to look at the medications that are listed in your chart. They might document that they have reviewed the medications, possibly by clicking a box to attest to having reviewed the medication list. They might not however, ask you to verify the medications that are actually in the chart. They may not verbally verify with you what is listed in the chart. It is important to clarify with them exactly what is written in the chart. Clarify what you are taking, how often you are taking it, what route you are taking it by, and make sure every medication that you are putting into or onto your body daily is on that list.

Advocacy Tip: Have your medication list and keep it up to date. If you were not given a printed list of your medications to review by the staff, hand your list (or a copy of it) to the clinician to ensure that they see the correct medications that you are taking. You can also ask the medical assistant or nurse to print out a copy of the medication list in your chart for your review.

Allergies/Adverse Reactions Revisited

We discussed the importance of your allergies and adverse reactions previously. However, it is important that you confirm with your clinician that the allergies and adverse reactions that are listed in your chart for that visit are accurate and up to date. Confirm not only what the allergens are, meaning what the things are that can cause a reaction, but it is important that they have the correct reaction listed. If you are ever in a life and death situation and you show up in an emergency department, the clinicians there may look at your list of allergies that are in the chart (something that can be done with sharing of some EMR information across facilities nationally). They might avoid giving you something that could be indicated or that could save your life because of your allergy list. If the only reaction that you get to a medication or an antibiotic is that it made you a little queasy, and it could save your life, then you can be given that medication and your clinician can help you with the queasiness. There is a difference between allergies and adverse reactions.

Advocacy Tip: Keep an updated list of your allergies and adverse reactions and take it with you everywhere.

Diagnosis Is in the Details

It is standard of care that everyone have a reason for their visit or a chief complaint documented as to why they are coming in. Let's return to the "toe pain" scenario. Your clinician has an understanding in this scenario that you have toe pain. After entering the room and sitting down, the clinician says, "I hear you have toe pain". You then begin elaborating on the toe pain and you both spend a lot of time on the toe pain. They examine you and go through the details of the toe pain. Based on what is already in the chart with your history, and whatever information they have gotten from you, they come up with a diagnosis. The diagnosis, believe it or not, is 90-95% derived based on the history you give. Let me repeat that. When clinicians make a diagnosis, they are taking a history and going through different diseases in their mind to try and gather data to either include those diseases on a differential diagnosis list (the list of possible diseases) or exclude them from the list. After they are done talking with you, they will then examine you and use the information from the exam to either confirm or exclude diseases that are on their differential diagnosis list. They order tests or imaging studies to confirm or exclude the remaining diseases on the list if needed. Most of the data that is used to come up with your diagnosis comes from the conversation that they have with you. So, it is very important that you take time to make sure that the communication is clear and accurate.

The Treatment Plan

Repetition, Clarification and Note Taking

Often patients do not repeat what has been told to them. It can be very helpful to repeat what has been told to you during the visit to confirm that you understand it. I recommend that you take notes so that you can look at them later and make sure that you did not misunderstand what was said at the visit. It is important that you not only understand what you should do, but for how long you should do it. In addition, ask about what you should do if things are not going according to the plan that was outlined for you.

Example:

You are prescribed a medication and go the pharmacy to pick it up. At the pharmacy, you find that the medication is too expensive for you or not available. You need to know whether it is okay if you don't have the medication.

- *Can you wait until the next visit?*

- *Do they need to call something else in?*

- *Maybe the medication is not available, and it is on backorder. Is it okay for you to wait for it to come in next week?*

- *Do you need to go to another pharmacy or get another drug so that you can start medication right away?*

These are some of the things that you need to have clear in your mind at the conclusion of your office visit.

Advocacy Tips:

- *Ask your clinician to write your instructions on your visit summary sheet.*
- *Ask how important it is that you start any new prescribed medications or treatments.*
- *Ask how soon you need to start any new medications or treatments.*

Follow Up

I often see communication errors regarding follow up. Let's say that you go in for an appointment and your blood pressure is a little elevated. The clinician says, "Okay, we should check that again next month". You go to make your appointment for follow up and the clinician is now booking out 3-4 months. It is important that you know if that is okay. If you have been told to follow up in a month, it is at that point that you need to communicate that you were told to follow up in 1 month. The person responsible for scheduling the appointment needs to speak to the clinician to make sure that the plan the clinician has laid out for follow up is adhered to. I have seen this issue quite frequently with specialist appointments.

If you are told to see a specialist for an appointment, it is important for you to know what time frame they want you to be seen in. It is important because if they think that you need to see a specialist urgently this week or next week at the latest, when the staff makes the appointment or gives you the information to make the appointment yourself, the specialist's office may say that the first available appointment with the specialist is in 3 months. You should be able to go back and say to your clinician that you can't get an appointment with a specialist until 3 months from now and your understanding is that they wanted you seen no later than next week. It is critical that you communicate and advocate for yourself so that you can make sure that you get the proper treatment in the proper time frame.

Things Left Unaddressed

Another issue that I often see in terms of communication errors are unaddressed issues and symptoms. Remember our toe pain scenario. You chatted with the medical assistant or nurse. They asked you why you were there. You said that you had toe pain to just get them in and get them out. They put that as the reason for the visit and the clinician comes in and talks about your toe pain. Now they begin to conclude the visit and say "well good, that's the plan for your toe pain. We will see you in a few months." They get up from their chair and head over to the door. As they grab the doorknob to leave, you say "Oh wait, I have a few more things to talk to you about." Now this is a problem because they may only have budgeted time to evaluate one issue. Ideally, they would have asked at the beginning of the visit, what things you wanted to talk about or why you were coming in and budgeted time accordingly. However, it is very easy to become sidetracked and spend time on things that they think are the only reason that you are there. This is problematic because now they are going to be behind schedule. Being behind schedule is a problem because physicians and other clinicians have become subject to patient satisfaction surveys. Surveys like Press Ganey and several others, ask patients questions to gauge their satisfaction. One of the questions that often gets asked is how long patients must wait for the provider in the exam room or the waiting room. These surveys can negatively impact the compensation of employed physicians and can have punitive consequences. As a result, the clinician running behind schedule can be problematic.

Failing to disclose concerns up front can be detrimental and possibly even lethal to you. Let's review a hypothetical list of problems that you brought in to discuss. Your list notes toe pain because you also have some arthritis in your toe. But you also have chest pain when you walk. When you go up a flight of stairs, it feels like an elephant is sitting on your chest. You have pain that goes into your left arm and into your jaw and you also are experiencing shortness of breath. It is likely that one of two things will happen once you tell your clinician that you have some other things that you would like to talk about as they are about to leave the room. They might say, "Okay", sit down, and hear what you have to say. Alternatively, they might say "I am sorry, our time is up for today and you will have to schedule another appointment". Now, if they come back and sit down, they will determine that you have a potentially life-threatening situation with heart disease and are having angina. They can then get you the appropriate testing or to see a cardiologist and hopefully, things will go well for you. If they tell you to make another appointment, you may find that the next appointment is three to four months out and you can't be seen sooner. If you walk out and do not communicate the urgency of the situation, or if you allow them to walk out and not have your issues addressed urgently, the consequences could be life threatening. It is important that you are mindful up front to present exactly what your needs are so that they can be met during the time that you are there.

Advocacy Tip: Make a list of your concerns and share the list at the beginning of your appointment. Acknowledge that you realize all the problems may not be able to be addressed at that visit, but that you want to ensure that any serious, potentially life-threatening problems are addressed.

CHAPTER NINE

After Visit Summary/Patient Portal

Given After Visit Summary Document or Patient Portal Invitation +/- information about recommended treatments/testing/medication/ follow up	**Communication Errors:** • Incomplete or Inaccurate Summary • Missing Information Needed for follow through • Importance of adhering to the plan • Contingency Plans (medication not covered/too expensive or specialist visit too far out)

Table 13

Once you have been evaluated, there is usually a plan of action discussed. Sometimes, they outline the plan on a visit summary or an after-visit summary. Many people don't read the visit summary sheet that is given to them. In some cases, the visit summary does not contain the important details of the plan that you need to successfully carry it out. Before the clinician leaves the exam room, most patients are given an after-visit summary or information about a patient portal that they can access via a code or by following specific steps. If you have not yet signed up for that patient portal, you will likely be given information about the recommended testing, treatments, what new medications to start, what medications to stop, and what the recommended follow up is on a paper summary. There are numerous potential communication errors that can occur in this process.

Inaccuracies and Discrepancies

Visit summaries can be incomplete or inaccurate. Someone may tell you one thing verbally but write something different on the summary. It is possible for them to be talking and writing something down on the summary during the visit and then change the plan later in the visit but forget to go back and change what they had written on the summary. It is very important that you review the visit summary to make sure that what it says on the summary is what you understand. That summary is also going to be in your chart and is what people believe you are following and doing. It is very important that it reflects what is actually happening. It might also be missing information that you need to follow through on the plan that has been prescribed for you. They may say, "I want to refer you to physical therapy", "I want you to see an endocrinologist", or "I want you to see a cardiologist", and the hope is that they have either given you the information or put a referral in. Sometimes however, there are so many things going on during the visit that the clinician is trying to address, they may forget to put the referral in, or they may forget to give you the information. You may walk out of the appointment and say "Oh, I know we talked about this, but I don't see anything on the visit summary about it". It is important that you verify everything that you believe to be a part of the plan.

Essentials

It is essential that you make sure that you have the information for how to get in touch with the specialist, and how to follow through with the referral. You need to make sure that you know how to do whatever it is that you are being told to do. Make sure that what you understand is happening between this visit and the next visit is what is being recommended to you. As I have said before, contingency plans are very important.

Contingency Plans

It is important to understand and communicate with your clinician about what the contingency plans are if the medication they have prescribed isn't covered, if the specialist visit is too far out, if the medication is too expensive or unavailable, or if there is a problem with whatever it is that they are asking you to do. In other words, if there is a problem, you need to understand what the contingency plan is.

We have just reviewed some of the communication errors that can happen with the after-visit summary. Being mindful that the potential for miscommunication exists even here, can help you avoid frustration and confusion.

Patient Portals

I often notice that patients do not sign up for the patient portals. They don't sign up because they do not think that they need to. Most patient portals have limited access to your medical records. Usually you have access to laboratory data and x-rays and can send and receive messages. Typically, you do not have access to telephone messages, office visit notes, consultation notes, and scanned documents. However, patient portals are actually a very important part of your medical record because it is where you can access and review a lot of data that is in the chart about you. Now there is also a movement called Open Notes[13] that allows you to be able to see the notes that have been written about your visit. I strongly encourage every patient to get those notes and review them. Make sure that what is said about you is what you understand and is accurate.

---

[13] https://www.opennotes.org/ (accessed November 28, 2018)

CHAPTER TEN

The Check-out

Closure

Now we move to the next portion of the office visit, which is check-out (Table 14). The check-out process can have many points for errors in communication to occur.

Communication Errors:

Check-Out ➡

- **Referrals and Referral Scheduling**
- **Follow up appointment**
- **Testing/Procedures**
- **Paperwork**

Table 14

Scheduling Referrals

Some of the errors that I find involve referrals and referral scheduling. Hopefully the person that is checking you out will schedule your appointment. Sometimes, as we discussed in the last chapter, that does not get done and the scheduling is left to you. This can be a problem because communication about when that appointment is needed doesn't always happen, and timing can often not reflect what the clinician desired. You may see a referral that you need to be seen in a week. The referral gets sent over to that department. Well, it turns out that there are no openings for an appointment in one week, so they book you an appointment in 3 months. They call or email you to tell you that you have an appointment in 3 months. This is a problem because you might be dead by the time you get to that appointment in 3 months. It is important that you make sure that the plan you have been given gets carried out.

Scheduling Primary Care Follow-up

Follow up appointments are another area where miscommunication errors occur. The clinician may tell you that they want to see you in 6 months, but you go to make that appointment and the staff tell you that the schedule is not open yet. You will have to call back. You go home and go on with your life, doing the things that you normally do. Later you remember that you needed to call back for an appointment in 6 months. You call and they are now booking out four to five months beyond the six months follow up that you needed. You finally go back in to be seen eleven months after your last visit. If there was something that your clinician wanted to check in six months, you are following up in almost double that amount of time. Something that was possibly a manageable problem before may now be a more serious life-threatening problem.

Advocacy Tip: Communicate the instructions that were given to you by the clinician. If the staff cannot assist you, speak directly to your clinician to verify that the new plan does not compromise your care.

Testing and Procedures

If you have been referred for a certain test or procedure, you may not have been given all the information required to schedule that appointment. The procedure or test may not be covered by your insurance or you may need a prior authorization for it. You may have been referred for an MRI and are claustrophobic (afraid of small enclosed spaces). It is essential that you verbalize any problems that you may have or any barriers that you are mindful of to having the procedures or testing that are recommended. It is very important that you have all the information needed to get that procedure or test done. You also need to know the desired timing for the testing. Ask when your clinician would like you to do the procedures or tests. Ensure that a test that they have ordered to follow up on something next week is not pushed out for months.

Advocacy Tip: Check and verify to ensure that you have complete understanding of what is required to complete the task. Review with your team the process you will follow by verbally repeating it to them.

Example: "I am being referred for a CAT scan. You would like me to have it done within _____ (days, weeks, months). I am to call (XXX-XXXX) and schedule the appointment.

Paperwork

Patients may have papers that they are given by the clinician to hand to the person at check-out. Sometimes everything that they need to know is not on the paperwork that is given to the person at check-out. Another scenario is that everything is not sent electronically to the person responsible for checking you out. It is important that you have a list in your own mind or a list on your own paper of what is being recommended for you so that you can double check that everything the clinician has recommended is being addressed and taken care of. Do not assume that it has been sent someplace and that it is being taken care of because that may not always be the case.

Advocacy Tip: Always take a notepad or paper to your appointments and take notes on what you are told and what you should do.

We have gone through the visit telephone game and as you can see, there are many places within the visit where communication and comprehension errors can occur. It is important as an advocate either for yourself or your loved ones, that you are mindful of where those errors can occur. It is also essential that you are proactive in making sure that the information contained within your record is accurate and that the information is clear.

In the next chapter, we will discuss the importance of reviewing your medical records.

CHAPTER ELEVEN

Reviewing Your Medical Record

The Details

The medical office visit is a complex process involving many people and the documentation of lots of information. Your medical record is a summary of what has occurred. As such, it is important to review your record for accuracy. Let's look at reasons to review your record and issues in some areas that you should be mindful of.

Miscommunication

- Can occur at *multiple points* during the visit

- Can *affect your diagnosis*. Ninety to ninety-five percent of the information used to diagnose disease comes from the history that is obtained from your chart and by speaking with you. Only approximately 2.5% of your diagnosis is based on your examination and approximately 2.5% from laboratory studies and testing.

- Can *cause incorrect information to be carried forward* from clinician to clinician as they enter information into the computer.

- Can *lead to misdiagnosis and inappropriate treatment and testing* if the diagnosis was derived from inaccurate information.

- Can *lead to death*. If you are misunderstood and an incorrect diagnosis is made based on that misunderstanding, treatment for the wrong diagnosis could be given and that misdiagnosis can lead to inappropriate testing, mistreatment, and even death.

Allergies

- Can be to *medications, food, or environmental allergens*

- Can range from being *mild to life threatening*

- Can *affect certain medications and procedures* in that some medications and procedures are contraindicated (should not be used) if you have certain allergies

- *EMRs and clinicians try to catch interactions.* They will use software or their clinical knowledge to be able to make sure that they are not prescribing something that is contraindicated based on either medications that you are taking, or allergies that you have. However, if your allergies are incorrect or not listed, clinicians may not catch a medication interaction or contraindication. This can result in significant injury, harm, or death.

Medication Errors/Omissions

- Applies to *both prescription and nonprescription* medications. Sometimes patients think that things that they buy over the counter are not significant. However, some medications that you buy over the counter are contraindicated with other medications that you may be being prescribed.

- Medications *can interact with each other*, sometimes in life threatening ways

- Clinicians *may not be aware of new or discontinued medications*. Maybe you were prescribed a medication and you stopped taking it because you did not like the way it made you feel. But you did not tell anyone, and they think that you are still taking it. It is important that you let them know that you are not on it or that you are having problems. Patients may see a specialist or a homeopathic doctor who does a lot with herbs and supplements. What you find is that Dr. H (the homeopathic clinician) may start new supplements or medications. Dr. H does not share the same electronic medical record with Dr. P, your primary care clinician. Dr. P will have no information that a new medication, supplement or herb has been started. Dr. P could as a result, prescribe something that could prove harmful or deadly because of a medication interaction. That is why it is important that ALL medications are accounted for on your medication list.

- Additional *medication may be prescribed that is similar to medications that you are already taking, leading to potential harm or toxicity*. This is especially true if you are using multiple pharmacies and no one has a complete medication list for you.

- *Some medications require monitoring* to ensure safety. I have seen some clinicians start a medication and it "falls off" or disappears from the medication list in the chart. It is very important that people are always aware that you are on a medication. You may be started on a medication and given six refills. You take the medication for six months but it "falls off" the list in the EMR. When you go in for a follow up, it might be easy for the clinician you are seeing to forget that you are on the medication since it does not appear on the medication list. It could be quite dangerous or even deadly for you take certain medications without it being monitored. These are the exceptions I hope, but I have seen in my over 26 years of practice, that these errors can occur.

Medical History Documentation Errors

- Can *follow you from provider to provider and from city to city*. Anything that is in your medical record whether accurate or not, will go with you when you have your records transferred to another clinician. If there are errors regarding your medical problems, errors regarding your habits or surgeries, those errors go with you. Know what is in your record. Make sure that it is accurate because the next person who takes care of you is likely going to believe what is in your chart, whether or not it is true. It is important to know that what is there accurately reflects the state of your health.

- Can cause you to *be denied life/disability insurance or pay higher premiums*. When you apply for insurance, they often ask for your medical records. Errors contained in the chart can affect whether you are insured and how much you end up paying for that insurance.

- Can *adversely affect your care if there is incorrect history in your chart*. I have talked about how history plays a role if someone accidentally clicks in the chart saying that you are a drinker, smoker and/or substance abuser. Maybe you have abdominal pain and you seek care, and someone had previously clicked that you had your gallbladder removed. Clinicians may start to rule diagnoses in, rule diagnoses out, or think of diagnoses that they ordinarily would not have thought of if your history had been correct. If you go in with gallbladder pain but your chart says that you have had your gallbladder removed and no one bothers to say, "Now I just want to confirm that you have had your gallbladder removed" allowing you to reply, "No, I have never had that surgery", it can adversely affect you. This is why it is so important that you verify all records for accuracy. The other issue is that these errors can go unnoticed for years. Try to identify these errors or discrepancies in your medical records as soon as possible because they may go unnoticed for years and be recognized only when a problem occurs.

Filing Errors

- Filing errors were much more common in my opinion when we had paper charts. Paper documents are still scanned into the medical record. Sometimes, the *scanning can be done into the wrong chart*. The way it usually works is that a document that did not originate within the same EMR system or that comes from a facility that doesn't feed the document automatically into that EMR, gets labeled with a sticker or a barcode that helps facilitate scanning. As with anything, user error is always possible. I have seen in some cases where a document that needed to be scanned in, had the wrong sticker placed on it. This caused it to be filed into the wrong chart. Scanned documents are sometimes scanned to parts of the chart that people may not review regularly. In some cases, things that are scanned in are not accessible to you when you access your patient portal. They also may not be readily visible to the clinician that is seeing you because they are filed in a portion of the chart, that they do not routinely look at when you come in for a visit. The problem with this is that when records are sent out or when someone else looks at the chart, they may find something in your chart, that is not information about you. It is only when someone says, "Oh I see you have had a stress test last year", and you say "No, I have never had a stress test", that they may then confirm the name on the document is not yours and the document itself is not about you. It is very important that for this reason, you know what your entire record contains.

- Documents will *become a part of your history*. Someone may do a chart review and update the chart and the problem lists in the chart. They may just look at the document that is in the chart without verifying that the name on the document that is in your chart is the same as your name and belongs to you. They may assume that the validation of the documents in your chart had been done by someone else. This can be problematic. I recommend that you review your history and if you hear that you have had a problem that you know you have never had or a procedure that you have never undergone, it is important that you ask where that information is coming from. Once a document is in the chart, some clinicians do not look at the name on the document. They look at what the document says. It is only when it is questioned that they will begin to verify that the information is correct. Therefore, it is critical to review this information.

- Dictation errors. Many facilities now use voice recognition software to transcribe the notes of clinicians. If you have ever tried dictating into your smartphone, you can already imagine what I am talking about. Things that are said do not get transcribed the way that you said them. This also happens with voice recognition software. What happens is that the clinician dictates one thing and the software transcribes something else. Clinicians have a limited amount of time to dictate a lot of information. Ideally, you would reread what you dictated and correct the errors. The problem is that the longer the text and the greater the amount of information that gets dictated, the less likely it is that you are going to be able to catch the errors. Your mind will fill in and your eyes will see what you were trying to say, not what is actually on the page. It is usually at a later point that the clinician will notice that there was an error. This is one of the challenges of proofreading your own work. When someone is doing a manuscript, someone else must proofread it. There needs to be a second set of eyes to help ensure accuracy because you are unlikely to catch all the errors. You know what you want to say, and your mind fills that in. These *errors may stay there until the next visit or they may stay there indefinitely*. These errors can range from errors with documentation of your examination to documentation errors with your history. Therefore, it is important that significant errors be addressed.

Now that I have explained why you should review your medical records, we will spend some time in the next chapter going over what steps to follow to obtain them.

CHAPTER TWELVE

Obtaining Your Medical Records

In order to help you be an advocate, I must spend some time talking about obtaining medical records both paper and electronic. You are legally (with rare exceptions) entitled to review your medical records and I highly recommend you look at the United States Department of Health and Human Services website:

https://www.hhs.gov/hipaa/for-individuals/medical-records/index.html

They have a vast amount of information regarding your rights and steps to obtain your medical records for yourself and/or for a deceased loved one.

I have listed some additional helpful websites below:

https://www.hhs.gov/sites/default/files/righttoaccessmemo.pdf

https://www.healthit.gov

https://www.healthit.gov/how-to-get-your-health-record

https://www.hhs.gov/sites/default/files/ocr/privacy/hipaa/understanding/consumers/consumer_rights.pdf

These sites also have information on privacy, HIPAA (Health Insurance Portability and Accountability Act of 1996). In general, you must fill out forms to access all of your medical records.

Patient Portal

You can access portions of your chart through the patient portal or through a portal that allows you to have access to your visit notes. You will have to sign up for access by following the instructions given to you by your healthcare team. Keep in mind that you may not have access to everything contained in your chart. Many patient portals have limited access to portions of the chart and no access to certain documents in your record.

Digital or Paper Copies

You will need to fill out a release of information or a records release request to have access to your complete medical records or to have a copy sent to someone for review. Usually they do not charge for you to have your records sent to a clinician, but this varies from institution to institution and provider to provider. There may be a charge if you ask for copies of your records to be sent to you for your personal review. In my consulting practice, I have rarely had my clients charged for records that have been sent to me. Most institutions can fax the record or send a secure link to the documents to be reviewed.

What If You Are Denied?

First, know your rights. Under HIPAA,[14] Health insurers and providers who are covered entities must comply with your right to:

- Ask to see and get a copy of your health records

- Have corrections added to your health information

---

[14] https://www.hhs.gov/hipaa/for-individuals/guidance-materials-for-consumers/index.html (accessed November 2018)

- Receive a notice that tells you how your health information may be used and shared

- Decide if you want to give your permission before your health information can be used or shared for certain purposes, such as for marketing

- Get a report on when and why your health information was shared for certain purposes

If you believe your rights are being denied or your health information isn't being protected, you can:

- File a complaint with your provider or health insurer

- File a complaint with HHS (US Department of Health and Human Services)

You should get to know these important rights, which help you protect your health information. You can ask your provider or health insurer questions about your rights. You may file a complaint if you are denied access or copies of your medical records with the U.S. Department of Health and Human Services Office of Civil Rights.

Do not allow yourself to be intimidated by the process of obtaining your records. Record requests are a standard part of the medical industry. Let your providers know that you are trying to be more involved in your medical care and want to make sure that you have a full understanding of how you can better participate in achieving the goals and plans you have discussed. In your healthcare, the only constant is likely to be you. Members of your healthcare team will come and go, but you will be with yourself every step of your journey. Be the expert on you. Know the who, what, why, where, when and how of your medical care. These details should help you be a better advocate for yourself.

CHAPTER THIRTEEN

Tips for Dealing with Errors

Some errors in documentation do not require urgent action. Examples are simple spelling, grammar and punctuation errors. As I mentioned previously, with voice recognition software or even typing, these errors will unfortunately occur. Correction of these errors will not likely change the quality of your medical care or lead to any harm.

Some errors require your immediate attention and you should notify your healthcare team as soon as you notice them. Examples are:

- Dates
- Medication information
- Medical History (Family, Personal, Social, Surgical)
- Diagnoses
- Results listed of tests that you know you have never had

- Incorrect Allergies
- Incorrect body part location on documentation of exam findings (right or left side)

If you find a significant error, you will want to let your healthcare team know:

- That there is an error in your record
- What the error is
- What the correct information is

Your healthcare team will then take steps to correct the error in the chart. If for some reason, they cannot correct the error, documentation can be filed noting that the error exists for future reference.

CHAPTER FOURTEEN

Teamwork

As you begin to advocate for yourself, it is important to remember that everyone is a valuable member of your team. Your clinicians have studied long and hard to help you. There are many factors that contribute to the experiences you have, and care that you receive when seeking medical care. Understand that most errors are not intentional but can result when systems and clinicians are strained.

Mutual respect, diligence, and teamwork will hopefully help you facilitate communication, have your concerns addressed, and your needs met. Remember, with few exceptions, you are likely the most knowledgeable about the topic of your health history. Healthcare requires teamwork. However, the central focus of the team must be you. The NP, DNP, MD, DO, PA, and the students come and go, but the one constant in your care is you. Therefore, you must be at the center of your care.

Healthcare requires teamwork but the leader must be YOU!

ABOUT THE AUTHOR

D r. Gina Cuyler was born in Panama, Central America. She immigrated to New York city with her mother at the age of 4 after her father died suddenly. After finishing High School, she received a full academic scholarship to New York University where she received a bachelor's degree in chemistry in 1988. She subsequently received her MD from the University of Rochester School of Medicine and Dentistry where she also completed her residency in Internal Medicine. Dr. Cuyler is board certified in Internal Medicine, a fellow of the American College of Physicians and a member of Alpha Omega Alpha Medical Honor Society. Dr. Cuyler is a National Academy of Sports Medicine Certified Personal Trainer and enjoys focusing on preventive care, wellness, and patient advocacy. An alumnus of University of Rochester School of Medicine and Dentistry, she remains active with teaching and holds a voluntary faculty appointment as a Clinical Assistant Professor of Medicine at the University of Rochester. Dr. Cuyler is owner and founder of Comprehension Internal Medicine PLLC, a direct to patient medical consulting firm. She has served as a faculty advisor for the GE National Medical Fellowship Program. She lives in Rochester with her husband and enjoys devoting time to her faith, family, and friends.

NOTES

Notes

Notes

Notes

Notes

Notes

Made in the USA
Middletown, DE
26 October 2020

22763567R00064